ANCIENT WISDOM

for

MODERN MINDS

T0166241

To Bronte with love.
May we continue to
grow in wisdom
and kindness.

ANCIENT
WISDOM
for
MODERN MINDS

JAMES CARLOPIO PhD

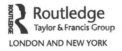

Routledge
Taylor & Francis Group

LONDON AND NEW YORK

First published 2007 by Goshawk Publishing

Published in 2016
by Routledge
2 Park Square, Milton Park, Abingdon, Oxon OX14 4RN
711 Third Avenue, New York, NY, 10017, USA

Routledge is an imprint of the Taylor & Francis Group, an informa business

National Library of Australia Cataloguing-in-Publication:

Carlopio, James R.
  Ancient wisdom for modern minds : a thinking heart for
  modern minds – words of insight into our selves.

  Bibliography.
  Includes index.
  ISBN 9780977574216.

  ISBN 0 9775742 1 0.

  1. Personal coaching. 2. Executive coaching.
  3. Self-perception. 4. Self-actualization (Psychology).
  5. Emotion. 6. Life skills. I. Title.

158.1

ISBN 13: 9780977574216 (pbk)

FOREWORD

When asked to review *Ancient Wisdom for Modern Minds*, I wasn't sure at first how I could help. At first it appeared to be a series of what I'd term 'quotes, blurbs, and affirmations'. This didn't make any sense, particularly because I understood the author to be a well-regarded academic from one of Australia's top business schools. I then had a flashback to the MA in business research work I did almost 10 years ago at MGSM, and the words 'hermeneutics' and 'deconstruction' popped-out! As a consequence, I understood what the author has set-out to achieve in presenting the wisdom of the ancients in a conversational coaching context for executives, HR managers, employees and reflective readers undergoing workplace and personal change.

Readers familiar with 'Positive Psychology' may regard the book as a qualitative data set for a meta-analysis, in an historical context, of four recurring themes, namely: (a) awareness of self and others; (b) life, death, health and happiness; (c) wisdom, communication and learning; and (d) achievement, goals and effort. The burgeoning Executive and Life

Coaching 'profession' is anchored within this paradigm. In presenting these quotes with references to other important areas in coaching psychology in the Introduction to each theme, James Carlopio shows us that coaching for personal improvement has been around since time-immemorial!

Considerable resemblances also exist between the ancient quotes (can we say advice?) and modern-day socio-cognitive constructs and techniques used in coaching psychology. In particular, coaching is based on the 'coaching conversation', itself grounded in the constructivist-narrative approaches used within Solution-Focused Brief Therapy.

Ancient Wisdom for Modern Minds has the potential to be one of the rare qualitative, post-modern (and humanistic) contributions to the epistemology of coaching psychology. With this in mind, I think *Ancient Wisdom for Modern Minds* will be a valuable coaching and educational tool – while providing very interesting insights to professional and lay readers alike!

Tom Crvenkovic
BA (Hons-Psych), MBA, MA (Business Research),
GradDipAppSci (Coaching Psych)
The Coaching Psychologist, Sydney - October 2006

CONTENTS

Foreword v

References viii

Preface ix

Part 1
Awareness of self and others 1

Part 2
Life and death, health and happiness 35

Part 3
Wisdom, communication and learning 69

Part 4
Achievement, goals and effort 91

Epilogue 111

Index 115

REFERENCES

Bernstein, E. (2006) Therapy that keeps on the sunny side of life; rising number of therapists focus on the positive instead of bad parents, other demons. The Wall Street Journal (Eastern Edition), September 26, D1.

Birkinshaw, J. & Gibson, C. (2004) Building ambidexterity into an organization. MIT Sloan Management Review, 45(4), 47-55.

Goleman, D., Boyatzis, R. & McKee, A. (2001) Primal leadership: The hidden driver of great performance. Harvard Business Review, 79(11), 42-51.

Latham, G. (2004) The motivational benefits of goal-setting. Academy of Management Executive 18(4), 126-129.

Lawson, W. (2004) The glee club. Psychology Today, 37 (1), 34.

Locke, E. (2004) Linking goals to monetary incentives. The Academy of Management Executive 18(4), 130-133.

Roach, D., Troboy, L. & Cochran, L. (2006) The effects of humor and goal setting on individual brainstorming performance. Academy of Business, 10(1), 31-36.

Sosik, J. & Megerian, L. (1999) Understanding leader emotional intelligence and performance. Group & Organization Management, 24(3), 367-390.

Turner, D. & Crawford, M. (1998) Change power. Business & Professional Publishing, Warriewood, NSW.

PREFACE

Ancient wisdom for modern minds

A Thinking Heart and a Feeling Mind
Words of Insight into Our Selves

A feeling heart is good;
A thinking heart is wise.

I like words. Millions of people use words every second of the day and give them very little, if any, serious thought as individuals. Yet somehow, collectively, these neglected individual words seem to work, as many of us carry out our daily routines, with their help.

As individuals some words are uniquely informative. When I do remember to pay some attention to them, they seem to provide me with insight into myself and into the human condition.

IX

The individual words in this book are compiled into phrases – thoughts, reflections and experiences voiced by ancient sages – as coaching conversations. Their wisdom creates a vibrant landscape populated with insights which help us through the emotions of change.

So, please come along with me on a journey experiencing the words in this book. We shall reflect on the wisdom of these ancient coaches with the intention of discovering what we can learn from them about our selves and our lives.

James Carlopio, PhD
Byron Bay – October 2006

AWARENESS OF SELF
AND OTHERS

AWARENESS OF SELF AND OTHERS

The two pillars of emotional intelligence are self-awareness as a precursor to learning better self-management, and awareness of others as a precursor to learning better management of others (Goleman et al., 2001; Sosik & Megerian, 1999). Self-awareness and awareness of others are also the keys to happiness, to personal satisfaction, and to successful relationships (Bernstein, 2006; Lawson, 2004). If we want to be successful and happy, we must take responsibility for our feelings, thoughts and behaviours. We must not blame others for our choices. Paradoxically, as we become more self-aware, we become less self-conscious – less worried about how we look to others and about what others think of us. This allows us to be more self-less and better able to work with, support and give to others. Self-awareness also provides us with a richer inner life and the ability to identify and focus on what really matters to us – the people we love. The quotes and reflections in this section are focused on topics such as personal responsibility and choice, giving and sharing, diversity, confidence and security, inner spirit, strength and awareness.

> Those who give hoping to be
> rewarded with honor are not giving,
> they are bargaining.

Philo, Egyptian philosopher (20 BC – 40 AD)

If we give with the expectation of return, or with the expectation of being recognised and rewarded for our generosity, it is not really giving. That is trading, purchasing or bargaining. Giving is self-less. There is no requirement for, or expectation of, return.

I give and I share. I gain satisfaction from the act of giving and sharing.

No man is hurt but by himself.

Diogenes of Sinope, Greek philosopher
(410 BC – 320 BC)

It is important for us to remember that no one can hurt our feelings. People can say and do what they like, and if you really do not believe what they say, it cannot hurt you. It is what we think and feel about ourselves that can hurt us. What others think and feel cannot hurt us unless we let it.

I am confident. I am secure. I choose my thoughts and my feelings.

To love is to expire.

Cleopatra, Egyptian Queen (69 BC – 30 BC)

In a sense, when we love fully, we give our Selves and our lives to some one or some idea, and we die or expire metaphorically. In another sense, when we love fully we, our Selves, cease to matter most. The object of our love becomes more important to us so we no longer matter as much and again, metaphorically we expire. We end in the sense that we stop being the most important thing in the world. This can be considered one of the truest, most mature forms of love, to be willing to consciously give your life for or to another.

I love deeply. I am capable of choosing to put someone else's needs before my own.

Beware the barrenness of a busy life.

Socrates, Greek philosopher (469 BC – 399 BC)

Busyness is a disease. It takes us away from the ones we love. It pulls us out of our inner selves and into the superficial outer world. It keeps us tired and lonely. It keeps us empty and numb. Only in stillness can we hope to find our Selves. Of course, we must make a living, go to school, take care of the kids and do the hundreds of things that are required to keep us healthy and happy on a daily basis. We also need time and space to rest and read, to think and to meditate, to be still and to play. We cannot fulfil our inner needs by staying outwardly busy.

I take time for my Self. I take time to be with the ones I love.

> As to marriage or celibacy, let a man
> take which course he will, he will be
> sure to repent.

Socrates, Greek philosopher (469 BC – 399 BC)

Relationships are difficult. So is living alone. The modern media, especially the entertainment media, tend to idealize relationships. Love is often portrayed in its magical 'happily-ever-after' phase. We must remember that relationships require energy, effort, discipline and determination. After the initial infatuation is gone, love and successful relationships are as much a matter of decision as they are a matter of feelings. Likewise, remaining celibate, or at least unmarried, also has its costs. Like most things in life, there are costs and benefits to all of our choices.

I create my reality. I am in love because I choose to be in love. I am in relationship because I choose to be in relationship. I am alone because I choose to be alone.

At high tide, fish eat ants; at low tide, ants eat fish.

Thai Proverb

In life, few things are exactly as they seem at first and with time everything changes. This is difficult for many of us to deal with. Some people try to ignore the fact. Others try and control who and what they can to bring a semblance of stability to their lives, even though it is illusory. Since many people find comfort in the familiar, we must remember that it is best to look for this stability within.

I am here. My essential spirit is eternal.

> How can you prove whether at this
> moment we are sleeping, and all our
> thoughts are a dream; or whether we
> are awake and talking to one another
> in the waking state?

Plato, Greek Philosopher (427 BC – 347 BC)

We do not know if our dreams are real or if what
we think is our reality is a dream. When we dream,
our dreams seem real to us at the time and we are
only aware they were dreams when we wake up
from them. Likewise, how do we know we are not
really dreaming when we think we are awake? Will
we someday wake up from what we thought at the
time was real to find out that this life too was
nothing but a dream? Is this what happens when
we die? Will we really wake up at the end of this
life and realise it was nothing but a dream within
our larger consciousness? Consciousness and
awareness are not well understood.

*My consciousness is a gift and I am thankful for
it. My awareness is a mystery and I revere it.*

> **Until you know yourself
> you will be distant from God.**

Rumi (14th century) Mystic poet

The very first step on the road to greater happiness, peace and contentment is self-awareness. The very first step on the road to greater achievement and success is self-awareness. The very first step on the road to spiritual enlightenment is self-awareness. Awareness is essential for all things good.

I am awareness of my Self. Every day I learn more about my Self. I grow to know my Self.

> Do not look back my friend no one
> knows how the world ever began.
> Do not fear the future, nothing is forever.
> If you dwell on the past or the future
> you will miss the moment.

Rumi (14th century) Mystic poet

While it is important to understand our personal and collective history, we would do well to remember that the past is not certain. Our individual and collective memories are fallible. While it is important to think about and plan for the future, we would do well to remember that every thing passes. Worrying about something that may or may not happen, wastes time and energy. It is most important to be conscious and aware of every moment. If we dwell on the past or the future, our lives will pass us by unnoticed.

I am conscious and aware. I understand the past and I learn from it. I plan for the future and I work toward it. I live now and cherish every moment of it.

11

> **True friendship is born out of love
> and is the water of life.**

Rumi (14th century) Mystic poet

> **A friend is a second self.**

*Aristotle, Greek critic, philosopher, physicist and zoologist
(384 BC – 322 BC)*

A true friend is one of the rarest and truest of blessings. Like a marriage, however, a friendship takes time, energy and effort. Friendships must be nurtured and protected. If they are well cared for, they are an abundant source of life, energy, solace and insight. Friends can say and do things that family and strangers cannot.

I nurture and care for my relationships.

> A child's life is like a piece of paper on which every passerby leaves a mark.

Chinese Proverb

Children are close to God. They are precious and vulnerable. Children are trusting and for many years they are completely dependent upon those around them. Parents, grandparents, extended family, friends, teachers, coaches, bus drivers and unknown passers-by in the streets all impact our children. Every remark and every gesture we make has an effect on them. They learn, through us, that they can, or cannot, trust and love. They learn that they are, or are not, special and wonderful, whole and capable, and safe and secure.

I speak and act with awareness and love, especially to children.

> The wine urges me on, the bewitching wine, which sets even a wise man to singing and to laughing gently and rouses him up to dance and brings forth words which were better unspoken.

Homer, Greek poet (800 BC – 700 BC), The Odyssey

There are two sides to intoxication and altered states of consciousness. The positive side is that sometimes an altered state of mind can help us to loosen up and see a different perspective. We sometimes feel more connected to others and are able to open up mystical doors. We can experience ecstasy, insight and great joy. Unfortunately, it is often the case that these experiences are either illusions, are short-lived or come at a great cost to ourselves and others. The negative side is that drugs and alcohol can cause great harm. Not only can they encourage us to say and do things we will regret later, they can cause devastating harm to individuals, families and our society.

I know my limits. I am conscious and clear.

14

> **A bad neighbour is a misfortune, as much as a good one is a great blessing.**

Hesiod, Greek didactic poet (~800 BC), Works and Days

Our neighbours and our community are critical to the quality of our lives. In our modern world, many of us find ourselves far away from our loved-ones and our extended families. When this occurs, our neighbours and our community become even more important to us. Cherish a good neighbour and involve yourself in your community. It will be good for you and good for our world.

I am connected to those around me. I count my good neighbours as a great blessing.

> The Way of Heaven is to benefit
> others and not to injure.
> The Way of the sage is to act but not
> to compete.

Lao-Tzu, Chinese philosopher (604 BC – 531 BC),
The Way of Lao-Tzu

Be aware of others, so we do no harm. It is important to be selfless sometimes and to work for the benefit of others. Be aware of Self, so we do what is right for us, not in comparison to external standards or expectations. It is important to be mindful of our Selves and to work for our own benefit.

I am aware of my Self. I am aware of others. I work for the benefit of my Self and of others.

> Above all else, guard your heart, for
> it is the wellspring of life.

King Solomon, Hebrew monarch (~1000 BC)

In our modern world, we tend to spend too
much time in our heads. We think, we worry, we
plan and we forget to feel. We tend not to spend
enough time in our hearts, from which wisdom,
spiritual transformation and most positive energy
arises.

*My heart is my consciousness. My heart thinks
and feels.*

> **The descent to Hades is the same from every place.**

Anaxagoras, Greek astronomer and philosopher (500 BC – 428 BC), from Diogenes Laertius, Lives of Eminent Philosophers

Just because someone is smart or beautiful or they have a lot of money, does not make them any better than anyone else. At work, the cleaners are people who are just as valuable, important and worthy of respect as the CEO. While it is true that each of these roles requires a different skill-set, there is nothing inherently better or worse in the people who occupy those roles, just because they occupy them. The road to ruin or to enlightenment is the same for everyone.

I am valuable. I am valued. I am worthy of love and respect.

> **A man may learn wisdom even from a foe.**

Aristophanes, Athenian comic dramatist
(450 BC – 388 BC)

Do not discount someone just because they are different from us or because our government and the news media have taught us to fear them. The modern person can learn a great deal from the so-called 'primitive' or 'barbarian'. There are many ways to view the world. Just because someone has a different worldview does not mean that they are ignorant or evil.

I honour and respect those who are different from me. I learn from difference.

> If you knew what I know about the
> power of giving, you would not let a
> single meal pass without sharing it in
> some way.

Buddha, Indian philosopher and religious leader
(563 BC – 483 BC)

Giving is as essential to mental health as a beating heart is to physical health. We often get so caught up in acquiring money and possessions for ourselves and our families that we forget that to give and to share is essential to life. If we only take, we eventually become barren and empty. If we only give, we also eventually become barren and empty.

I give and I receive. I receive and I give.

> We cannot control the evil tongues
> of others; but a good life enables us
> to disregard them.

Cato the Elder, Roman orator and politician
(234 BC – 149 BC)

We have been taught that the causes of our problems are usually other people and circumstances. It follows, therefore, that we have also come to expect that the solutions to our problems are to be found somewhere outside of ourselves as well - in others and/or in changing circumstances. This is a fallacy. When we are conscious, aware, balanced and whole we realise we cannot be hurt by the words of others unless we believe them. We have the power to disregard them. We can then be healthy and happy and we can choose to disregard the 'evil tongues' of others.

I have all that I need within my Self. I can
protect my Self from unwanted words, thoughts
and energy from others.

> Be sure that it is not you that is mortal, but only your body. For that man whom your outward form reveals is not yourself; the spirit is the true self, not that physical figure which can be pointed out by your finger.

Cicero, Roman author, orator and politician
(106 BC – 43 BC)

Our essential inner spirit is the wellspring of life, not our physical forms. The egg yoke is the source of life for us all. It is pure potential. From this core, we grow and take flight. Your yoke, Yoga or Yogi does not have to be an individual that you worship. Your Yoga is your essential place, your union, where you join and become one. Find your Yoga and exercise it. Through exercise, it will grow. You will come to realise that you are not that physical figure which can be 'pointed out by your finger'. You are Yoga, spirit and pure potential.

I am Yoga. I am spirit. I am pure potential.

> In these matters the only certainty is
> that nothing is certain.

Pliny the Elder, Roman savant (23 AD – 79 AD)
Natural History

We must learn not to expect certainty. While we
can make plans and set goals, and it is good to do
so, we must also remember that the universe is
not here solely to fulfil our wishes and desires. We
must learn to accept, and to plan for, the fact of
uncertainty in our world and in our lives.

I am confident in my choices. I am flexible
enough to realise that while nothing is guaranteed,
I stand firm in my convictions.

Men willingly believe what they wish.

Julius Caesar, Roman political and military leader (100 BC – 44 BC) Commentarii de Bello Gallico

It sometimes seems better to believe what is easy to believe, than to think for our selves. Do not allow yourself to fool your Self. What you read in newspapers or see on the television is not always true. It does not have to be believed. It may be the truth from someone's perspective, but it is not necessarily the objective truth, nor is it necessarily what you have to believe. Remember that if you believe something, you are choosing to believe it.

I am conscious and aware. I choose what I believe.

> What is food to one, is to others
> bitter poison.

Lucretius, Roman poet and philosopher (99 BC – 55 BC)
De Rerum Natura

We are each unique in some ways. Do not assume that what is good for someone else, will necessarily be good for you. We each must make up our own minds about what nurtures and feeds us. It frequently seems easier to copy and to assume that the diet or the philosophy or the guru that works for someone we know, will work for us. Fads come and go, but we must remain conscious and aware of what works and does not work for us. While there is nothing wrong with trying 'the latest …', we must remember that we are the final arbiters of what nurtures us.

I am flexible and willing to try new things, and I
am aware of what is good for my Self.

Men are only clever at shifting blame from
their own shoulders to those of others.

Titus Livius, Roman author and historian (59 BC – 17 AD)

Often in our lives, people say and do things that
seem to cause us pain. Instead of blaming others for
our problems, if we take responsibility for our
thoughts, feelings and reactions, we retain a sense of
power and influence in our lives. Taking responsibility means we do not have to blame. When we
take responsibility we are present and aware, we do
what we say we are going to do, we are fully present
and aware and, therefore, response-able – that is, we
are able to respond to what is actually happening to
us moment to moment. This gives us choices. When
we react to triggers, such as what someone else says
and does, or when we blindly react to patterns from
our past, we give away our power and our ability to
respond consciously.

*I am at choice. I can choose my response to what
others say and do, and to what goes on around
me. I am response-able … I am able to respond.*

> Cherish that which is within you and
> shut out that which is without.

Chuang-Tzu, Chinese philosopher (369 BC – 286 BC)

It is from our inner strength and valour, that our true value and worth is determined. Our value in life is not determined by external things such as how much money we make. Our value in life is determined by our inner strength, our values and our convictions. Our value comes from what we think, feel, say and do. We must cherish and value our inner selves and not become too distracted by or focused on that which is on the outside.

I have value. I am strong and worthwhile. I am valuable.

> Flow with whatever is happening and
> let your mind be free. Stay centered
> by accepting whatever you are doing.
> This is the ultimate.

Chuang-Tzu, Chinese philosopher (369 BC – 286 BC)

When faced with crisis or emergency many of us
split - we panic, get thrown off balance and we
split or separate from our Selves. Those of us who
can handle crises, and seem to stay calm and
collected in the face of a problem or emergency,
do so by staying centered within ourselves, by
staying connected to, conscious and aware of our
Selves. To stay centered, we need to continually
be aware of what we are doing and accept it.

*I am centered. I am aware of and accepting of
what I am doing. I am connected to, conscious and
aware of my Self no matter what is happening
around me.*

> No one can give you better advice
> than yourself.

Cicero, Roman author, orator and politician
(106 BC – 43 BC)

We know what we need to do. When we make a decision, however, we cut off certain possibilities. That is why decisions are sometimes difficult to make. When we decide, we actually have to give up, and close down, certain possibilities. Although it is true that decisions are in some ways an ending, they are also a beginning. When we choose a certain path, and make a decision, we open up to the vast possibility that is offered by the choice. Decision-making becomes easier when we remember both of its sides – cutting off and opening up. We can then balance the loss with what we gain and we need little advice from others.

I know what I need to do and when I decide
to do it, I open up to the possibilities that
are offered.

He who knows others is wise;
He who know himself is enlightened.

Lao-Tzu, Chinese philosopher (604 BC – 531 BC)
The Way of Lao-Tzu

When we act automatically, without self-thinking or conscious thought, we are machine-like, not connected to our hearts and our Higher Selves. We act in response, from force of habit, out of old patterns that frequently no longer serve us. As we grow and become more conscious and aware of who and what we are, we become less automatic, less machine-like, and more alive. The more we know about our Selves the more we are at choice and the less we are unconscious, acting and thinking from old patterns without awareness.

I am conscious and aware of my-self.
I am at choice.

> Unless you believe, you will not
> understand.

Saint Augustine, Carthaginian author and church father
(354 AD – 430 AD) De Libero Arbitrio

When we believe, we see above and beyond the
commonplace and we adhere to it. In other words,
when we believe we see something extraordinary
and we take it as real ... we believe it. In order to
understand and see what is true for us and within
us, we must believe in ourselves. In order to achieve
anything in this word, we must believe that we can.
In order to receive love, we must believe in it. In
order to know truth, we must believe in it. In order
to see beauty, we must believe in it. In order to live
peacefully, we must believe in it. It is good to
believe.

I believe. I see above and beyond the commonplace
and it is real.

31

> What the superior man seeks is in himself; what the small man seeks is in others.

Confucius, Chinese philosopher and reformer
(551 BC – 479 BC)

We sometimes think that in order to have a proper or suitable place in this world, and to belong, we must completely go along with what others want. We believe we will finally belong, be loved and fit in when we follow the crowd, or when we do what our parents or society seems to want us to do. We will never belong, be loved or fit in, however, by blindly going along with or following the wishes of others. We will only truly belong, and find our proper and suitable place in the world, if we completely go along with and follow our Selves and what we know to be right and true.

I belong. I have a proper and suitable place in this word ... where I am.

It is in the character of very few men
to honour without envy a friend who
has prospered.

Aeschylus, Greek tragic dramatist (525 BC – 456 BC)
Agamemnon

As iron is eaten away by rust, so the
envious are consumed by their own
passion.

Antisthenes, Greek philosopher (444 BC – 371 BC)

Jealousy is a complex, often ignored emotion. It
is usually thought of as being negative, as in spite
and envy. Jealousy also has a positive side. When
we aspire to be like someone, we see her/him as
a positive role model. This is positive jealousy. In
this way, we can honour another without envy. It
helps us to stretch, to learn and to grow.

I recognise, honour and am inspired by the
achievements of others.

> The softest things in the world over-
> come the hardest things in the world.
> Through this I know the advantage
> of taking no action.

Lao-Tzu, Chinese philosopher (604 BC – 531 BC)
The Way of Lao-Tzu

> A happy life consists in tranquillity
> of mind.

Cicero, Roman author, orator and politician
(106 BC – 43 BC)

When we are being, not doing, we transform into
our Higher Selves. We are then able to see above
and beyond. Just being, not doing, is an important
part of our existence. Meditation, relaxation, Yoga
and practices that take us inward and help us be
still, allow us to better see both inward and outward
and to become more conscious and aware.

I see inward and outward, above and beyond.
I am being, not doing.

LIFE AND DEATH,
HEALTH AND HAPPINESS

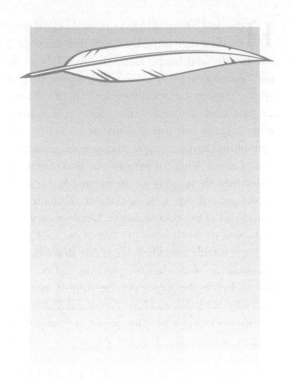

LIFE AND DEATH,
HEALTH AND HAPPINESS

How do I or should I live? How do I deal with the fact that someday I will die? How do I stay healthy and happy along the way? These are the core issues of life. How we deal with and answer these questions forms the core of who we are and how we deal with others, as it colours every aspect of our experience of life. We continually make choices and we tell ourselves stories about what happens in our lives. Until we realise how thoroughly we are the architects of our experience of our lives, we are at the mercy of others and of the circumstances. Until we confront and come to terms with the fact of our mortality, we cannot truly live. Until we realise that what we tell ourselves and what we put into and do with our bodies, is the major determinant of how we feel, what we think and how happy and healthy we are, we are living a lie. The quotes and reflections in this section are focused on topics such as integrity, forgiveness, abundance, anger, balance, passion, enthusiasm, respect, health and well-being.

> If thou suffer injustice, console
> thyself; the true unhappiness is in
> doing it.

Democritus, Greek philosopher (460 BC – 370 BC)

This is one of the hardest lessons for anyone to learn. When we are wronged, it seems natural to feel unhappy or injured. Why not? We did nothing wrong. We did not deserve it. We feel justified, often righteous in our indignation. What is so hard to see is that when someone hurts another, they do so out of their own hurt and they further hurt themselves in so doing. When we are wronged, therefore, we have a choice. We can feel victimised, we can get angry and we can even look for revenge, none of which does us any good. The alternative is that we can consider how fortunate we are, that we are not the one who has done the harm. In this way we show understanding and are forgiving. We do not become a victim and we suffer less harm.

I choose how I think, feel and react. I choose to think, feel and react in ways that serve me.

> **Everyone has a doctor in him or her;
> we just have to help it in its work.**

Hippocrates, Greek physician (460 BC – 377 BC)

When we are healthy, whole and happy we feel holy, and when we are holy we feel healthy, whole and happy. We cannot be whole (or healthy, happy and holy) without some semblance of balance between our rational, reasonable, logical side and our spiritual, emotional, intuitive side. This is how we help ourselves heal. Eating well helps our inner doctor. Being positive in our thoughts helps our inner doctor. Doing the right thing helps our inner doctor. Exercise helps our inner doctor. Forgiveness helps our inner doctor. A balance and harmony between work and family, between thinking and feeling, between planning and doing – these things enable our inner doctor to keep us well or, when we loose this balance and become unwell, regaining this balance helps us to restore health.

I am holy … healthy, whole and happy. My inner doctor has all it needs to make me and keep me well.

> Words are the physicians of the
> mind diseased.

Aeschylus, Greek tragic dramatist (525 BC – 456 BC)
Prometheus Bound

We are our word. Because we say it, it is true. We can make ourselves sick, by what we say to ourselves. We can heal ourselves, by what we say to ourselves. If we continually think we are happy and well, we are more likely to be so. The power of our intentions and of the words that we speak is inestimable.

I say what I mean and I mean what I say, and so saying it, it is true.

> **Forget injuries, never forget kindnesses.**

Confucius, Chinese philosopher and reformer
(551 BC – 479 BC)

When we absolve ourselves, or someone else, of guilt, for example, we are free from it. We free ourselves, and them from the chains that bind us and we create a new freedom into which greater life and energy can flow. It is forgiveness and absolution that sets us free.

I absolve myself and those who have harmed me.
I am free to live and to love.

> ### No single thing abides, but all things flow.

Lucretius, Roman poet and philosopher (99 BC – 55 BC)

> ### Everything flows.

Heraclitus, Greek philosopher (535 BC – 475 BC)

Affluence is the abundant flow, the giving and taking of the energies in life. When the energies of life are flowing abundantly we find we are affluent as we have enough of what ever we need in our lives.

I am affluent. I am abundant. I am in the flow of life and have enough of what ever I need in my life.

> Anger so clouds the mind, that it
> cannot perceive the truth.

Cato the Elder, Roman orator and politician
(234 BC – 149 BC)

> When anger rises, think of the
> consequences.

Confucius, Chinese philosopher and reformer
(551 BC – 179 BC)

When we are angry, we are constricted. This may
result from injury or mistreatment, but anger
negatively impacts on our experience of our
lives. The energy of life cannot flow to us, from
us, or within us when we are angry. Anger kills
happiness and life as it restricts, constricts and
narrows our perceptions and feelings.

I am free of anger and my life and my
energy flows.

> **The goal of life is living in
> agreement with nature.**

Zeno, Greek philosopher (335 BC – 264 BC)
from Diogenes Laertius, Lives of Eminent Philosophers

We must strive to live in harmony with our world. Of course, we are all now aware that we must do things such as reduce our wastes and our use of carbon-based fuels, but we must also live in harmony with others and with ourselves. We must give to the earth, and to others, as much as we take so we are in agreement with nature and are balanced and sustainable.

I am in balance. I am complete, whole and satisfied. I am living in agreement with nature.

> Indeed, what is there that does not
> appear marvellous when it comes to
> our knowledge for the first time?
> How many things, too, are looked
> upon as quite impossible until they
> have been actually affected?

Pliny the Elder, Roman savant (23 AD – 79 AD)
Natural History

Many things seem impossible until we do them.
When we resolve to be the best we can, or to do
the impossible, we are going past what we have
been considering as normal and 'doable'. When
we resolve to be or become the best, we go above
and beyond our limits, reaching toward our goals,
toward happiness, fulfilment and our Higher
Selves to become all that we can be.

I am continually becoming, going and seeing
beyond my boundaries toward happiness
and fulfilment.

Intellectual passion dries out sensuality.

Leonardo da Vinci, Italian engineer, inventor, painter and sculptor (1452 – 1519) The notebooks

While awareness and self-knowledge are paramount, sometimes over intellectualising or excessive thinking and worry can dry up the pleasure in life. When we use all of our senses, and are sensual, we are passionate and enthusiastic; we are full of life, delight and excitement. That is why enthusiasm is also defined as supernatural inspiration or possession, inspired prophetic or poetic ecstasy, and religious frenzy.

I am passionate. I care deeply. I am enthusiastic, spiritual and full of life, light and excitement.

> Do not set foot on the path of the
> wicked or walk in the way of evil
> men. Avoid it, do not travel on it;
> turn from it and go on your way.

King Solomon, Hebrew monarch (~1000 BC)

We are often influenced by the behaviour of
others and by the situations in which we find
ourselves. Our behaviour is significantly influenced
by our physical and social surroundings. When
we recognise that a certain place, course of
action, person or group of people is not right, nor
good for us, we must have the courage to walk
away.

*I am goodness and love. I surround myself with
goodness and love.*

> Though boys throw stones at frogs in
> sport, the frogs do not die in sport,
> but in earnest.

*Bion of Phlossa, Greek bucolic (pastoral) poet (~100 or
150 BC) from Plutarch's Water and Land Animals*

There is often a world of difference between what
we intend and what actually happens or what is per-
ceived by another. Our internal witness helps us
become aware of who we are and how we are in the
world. It helps us to distinguish between what actually happens and what we intend. Our witness allows
us to see and to know ourselves. We access our witness by dividing our attention so that we are 100%
conscious of our actions, feelings and thoughts in the
moment, and yet still aware of what is happening
around us, using some portion of our consciousness
watching ourselves. It is possible to do this because it
is possible to be more than 100% in this way. This is
possible because our consciousness is infinite.

*I am a witness. I am aware and conscious of what
I do, what I intend and what actually happens.*

47

> He harms himself who does harm to
> another, and the evil plan is most
> harmful to the planner.

Hesiod, Greek didactic poet (~800 BC) Works and Days

Revenge, born of anger and the need for retribution, hurts the vengeful. Revenge does not right the wrong that has been done and never helps the vengeful feel better in the long run. If a wrong is acknowledged it is easier to heal it. Confronting someone who has done you wrong, expressing your feelings and letting them know the consequences of their wrong-doing is not revenge, it is wisdom. It helps you to recognise and express your emotions, to gain closure and to begin the healing process. Forgiveness is the goal.

I have a right to my emotions. I have a right to be treated fairly and with respect. I also have a duty to treat others fairly and with respect.

I am sure the grapes are sour.

Aesop, Greek slave and author (620 BC – 560 BC)
The Fox and the Grapes

Our expectations are powerful forces in our lives. What we expect to happen often will happen. Our expectations create our reality. Both consciously and unconsciously our expectations affect our behaviour and the behaviour of others. If we expect the worst to happen, quite often it will. If we expect the best of ourselves and of others, equally often it will.

I expect the best of myself and of others.

From the end spring new beginnings.

Pliny the Elder, Roman savant (23 AD – 79 AD)
Natural History

Life is a cycle. Everything that lives, grows, matures and ends. Everything that begins eventually ends. While it is normal and healthy to mourn these endings, it is also heartening to remember that within these cycles every ending heralds a new beginning. When we move house, we start living somewhere new. When we end a job, we start another job or another phase in our lives. When a plant or flower ends its life, from its seeds springs new life. These are immutable laws of the universe. There are no exceptions. Therefore, it must be that when our life ends a new beginning springs forth.

I am part of the cycle of life. I trust that from every ending springs forth new beginnings.

> Man perfected by society is the best of all
> animals; he is the most terrible of all when
> he lives without law, and without justice.

Aristotle, Greek critic, philosopher, physicist and zoologist
(384 BC – 322 BC)

Boundaries are critical. They provide security and protection. Boundaries let us know what is and is not acceptable. Boundaries help keep us safe and help protect us from others and from ourselves. With children, for example, a set bed-time or an established set of chores that must be completed provides limits within which they can learn discipline and grow. Of course they will push those boundaries, but staying firm provides stability and ensures opportunities for discussion, negotiation and learning. As adults, setting boundaries that we will not let others cross (e.g., not letting another take advantage of you, keeping work separate from home) is a manifestation of respect for the Self.

I respect my Self and others as I set and maintain
appropriate and clear boundaries.

United we stand, divided we fall.

Aesop, Greek slave and author (620 BC – 560 BC)

Many people today feel isolated and disconnected in many ways. Thousands of us live in close physical proximity with thousands of others (e.g., in apartments and on trains and busses), and yet we feel isolated and lonely. Neighbours are strangers. Adjacent countries are mortal enemies. All of this division inevitably leads to the fall of us all.

We are one people. We are one planet.

> When we see men of a contrary character, we should turn inwards and examine ourselves.

Confucius, Chinese philosopher and reformer (551 BC – 479 BC)

> You are my face, small wonder that I cannot see you.

Rumi, Persian mystic poet (14th century)

Often what we like least in others is abundant within ourselves. Likewise, what we like most in others is abundant within ourselves. Psychologists refer to this as projection – we often unconsciously attribute our own attitudes, feelings or suppositions to others. Profound learning can take place when we recognise aspects of another's personality in ourselves that we do not like. Others often act as a mirror. It is easier to see these faults in others than in ourselves.

I own and take responsibility for my attitudes, feelings and assumptions.

It is a true saying that 'One falsehood
leads easily to another'.

Cicero, Roman author, orator and politician
(106 BC – 43 BC)

Hateful to me as the gates of Hades
is that man who hides one thing in
his heart and speaks another.

Homer, Greek poet (800 BC – 700 BC), The Iliad

Lies are traps. Lies are a slippery slope, for once
you start down their path their accumulated
momentum becomes a powerful force difficult to
alter. If you are an intelligent or accomplished liar,
you may be able to fool many people. The one
person who counts the most, however …
yourself, always knows the falsehood and cannot
be fooled. When we lie it causes dissonance in our
spirit, mind and body and we pay an awful price.

I speak the truth.

54

> **Our food should be our medicine.**
> **Our medicine should be our food.**

Hippocrates (460 BC – 377 BC) Greek physician

We are what we eat … literally. Our physical bodies, all of our organs and tissues, are literally made from what we consume. Our bodies completely replace all of our tissues and cells every one to seven years. The cells of our eyes replace themselves every two days. The intestinal lining is replaced every five to 30 days. Liver cells regenerate every 6 weeks. So, if we feed ourselves negative thoughts and processed, artificial chemical-filled foods, that is all that is available and it is used to produce and reproduce our cells, tissues and our organs. If we want to heal our body, we must feed it positive thoughts, clean water and healthful foods.

Every cell in my body grows healthy and strong.

Walking is man's best medicine.

Hippocrates (460 BC – 377 BC) Greek physician

Exercise is essential to mental and physical well-being. Studies consistently illustrate that exercise can help protect us from heart disease and stroke, some forms of cancer, high blood pressure, diabetes, obesity, back pain, osteoporosis, and more. It can also help reduce depression and anxiety, improve psychological well-being and help us to better manage stress. If you exercise your mind, it stays flexible and capable. If you exercise your body, it stays flexible and capable. There is no substitute and there is no excuse justifiable for not exercising. We must do what ever form of exercise we can do.

I regularly exercise my mind and my body. I am physically and mentally flexible and capable.

> A wise man should consider that health is the greatest of human blessings, and learn how by his own thought to derive benefit from his illnesses.

Hippocrates, Greek physician (460 BC – 377 BC)
Regimen in Health

Illness is a signal to us that something is wrong. If we think evil, poisonous thoughts, they eventually will harm our bodies. If we are stressed constantly, our body will eventually pay a price. If we do not eat well, or if we smoke, drink to excess or do not get enough exercise, we will not have optimal health. So when we are ill, we need to think about what our body is telling us. When we are ill we must consider what we can learn about what we are thinking and doing that is, or is not, serving our best interests in the long run.

I listen to my body, mind and soul. I nurture and love my body, my mind and my soul.

> **The great man is he who does not lose his child-heart.**

Mencius, Chinese philosopher (371 BC – 289 BC)

In our modern world, we spend far too much time being serious, especially at work. Even as children, we are becoming more serious earlier. We are expected to be able to read, for example, by the time we are age four or five. As parents we start seriously 'working on' our children even before they are born expecting them to grow up and achieve. While there is nothing wrong with the lifelong pursuit of achievement and learning, we must remember to take regular and significant periods of time 'off' for rest, relaxation and recreation.

I am able to have fun and to relax.
I play every day.

> Humor is the only test of gravity, and gravity of humor; for a subject which will not bear raillery is suspicious, and a jest which will not bear serious examination is false wit.

Aristotle, Greek critic, philosopher, physicist and zoologist
(384 BC – 322 BC)

Whatever problem or disaster has befallen us, looking for the humour within it can bring us perspective and help us to better deal with it. It is also important for us to remember that we often hide hard-to-express truths in humour. It makes it safer to express ourselves as we can always say we were 'just kidding' or 'not serious' as it was 'just a joke.' Unfortunately, this is not an effective way to communicate. If something important needs to be said, while it may be difficult to say and we may feel uncomfortable saying it, if we want to solve the problem or clear up the issue it must be discussed.

I keep things in perspective. I keep the bigger picture in mind. I am able to say what needs to be said.

The Gods too are fond of a joke.

Aristotle, Greek critic, philosopher, physicist and zoologist
(384 BC – 322 BC)

Our lives are full of ironic and paradoxical situations. We can let them anger and frustrate us. We can let them depress us and we can become jaded and cynical. Alternatively, we can learn to live with them. We can accept them as the jokes of the Gods and laugh along with them. The choice is ours.

I choose to see light and humour in my life.

> Among all men on the earth bards
> have a share of honour and
> reverence, because the muse has
> taught them songs and loves the race
> of bards.

Homer, Greek poet (800 BC – 700 BC), The Odyssey

> Please God, offer honey to musicians
> who bring us such joy!

Rumi (14th century) Mystic poet

There is a need for the arts in our lives. One of the best ways to nourish our Selves is through art, music, poetry, story-telling and other creative arts. The arts help expand our minds, bodies and spirits and are as necessary to a full life as food and water.

I am creative. I exercise and nurture my creativity.

> Dictatorship naturally arises out of democracy, and the most aggravated form of tyranny and slavery out of the most extreme liberty.

Plato, Greek Philosopher (427 BC – 347 BC)

Many of us who have always lived with freedom, forget that not everyone else on our earth does and that for most of human history very few have. Let us not take such a rare gift for granted lest we loose it. We must also be mindful of the modern paradox of freedom. In some places, people are so free that we have to live behind bars in our homes and in gated communities to protect ourselves, and thus, paradoxically, we have drastically limited freedom. Some people are afraid to go out on to their streets at night. Have we taken freedom so far that is has come back to haunt us?

I appreciate the gifts I have been given in this life.

> As a well-spent day brings happy
> sleep, so life well used brings
> happy death.

Leonardo da Vinci, Italian engineer, inventor, painter and
sculptor (1452 – 1519)

When we fear death, it is often that we fear that
we have not yet fully lived. Many of us fear death
because we have not done all that we want to do
or have not said all that we need to say. We do not
fear death as much as we fear not be here. In our
modern world we often spend two-thirds of our
life at work, commuting to and from work and
sleeping. That leaves only one-third of our lives
for everything else including what most of us
would say are the most important parts – family,
friends, travel, recreation, etc. We need to live, so
we will not fear death.

I say what needs to be said. I do what is most
important to me. I spend my time on the people
and pursuits that matter to me most.

> Deafened by the voice of desire you
> are unaware the beloved lives in the
> core of your heart. Stop the noise and
> you will hear his voice in the silence.

Rumi (14th century) Mystic poet

In our modern, materialistic world, many people believe that our material possessions will bring us happiness. When I get a new car, then I'll be happy. When I get a bigger house or a plasma flat-screen TV, then I'll be content with my life. For those of us fortunate enough to have the basic survival essentials in life (food, water and a safe place to live), it rarely happens that the acquisition of material possessions brings long-lasting peace and contentment. When we stop the internal chatter and still the media-feed frenzy of material desire, we can begin to become more self-reflective and aware of our Selves.

I choose to be happy. I am content and peaceful.

> Don't get lost in your pain. Know
> that one-day your pain will become
> your cure.

Rumi (14th century) Mystic poet

Our emotional and physical pain is there for a reason. Pain is a signal that something is wrong. Our spirit, mind and body use pain to get our attention.

If we get lost in our pain and become less conscious, we cannot learn what it has to teach. By attending to our pain, we can find its source and start the healing process. If we do not do this, we will continue to recreate the problem in our lives over and over again until we either attend to it or run out of days.

I am aware of my pain. I can find the source of my pain, expose it to the light of day, and heal it.

Beauty is a short-lived tyranny.

Socrates, Greek philosopher (469 BC – 399 BC)

We cannot stay young, healthy and physically beautiful all of our lives. Of course, we can try to remain as healthy and as active as we can, for as long as we can, and this will help us retain our youth and beauty for as long as possible, but to be a slave to external notions of physical beauty is foolishness. What can be continuously developed and maintained all of our lives is our inner beauty. Inner peace, tranquillity, balance and harmony will radiate outward as a beauty greater than any cosmetic beauty.

I am peaceful and balanced. I am tranquil and harmonious. I am beauty.

> What is lawful is not binding only on
> some and not binding on others.
> Lawfulness extends everywhere,
> through the wide-ruling air and the
> boundless light of the sky.

Empedocles, Greek philosopher (490 BC – 430 BC)

Double standards are common as people often can
see the world only from their point of view and
have an inflated sense of their capabilities. For
example, 'It is OK that I exceed the posted speed
limits while driving because I am a good driver.
Most others, however, should stay under the speed
limits'. Interpersonally we also often apply double
standards. It is OK when I do not clean up after
myself in the kitchen or drop clothing around the
house because I am in a hurry or I will do it later.
Of course, if anyone else were to do the same, that
would not be acceptable.

I see the truth. I apply the truth equally to all.

> Healing is a matter of time, but it is sometimes also a matter of opportunity.

Hippocrates, Greek physician (460 BC – 377 BC), Precepts

With most 'normal', every-day physical injuries, healing occurs naturally with time. With psychological and emotional trauma, however, the mere passage of time does little to heal. Life, however, will regularly provide opportunities for us to look at our issues and to deal with them, but we must recognise and seize these opportunities. If we do not, we will be doomed to continually re-experience these patterns and the problems they bring.

I recognise the problems I cause myself. When opportunities for forgiveness and healing come my way, I am aware of them and I use them.

WISDOM,
COMMUNICATION,
AND LEARNING

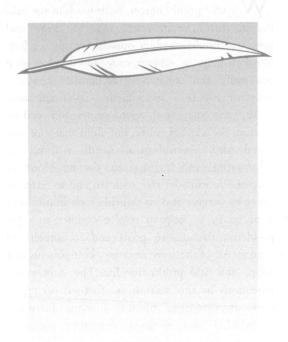

WISDOM, COMMUNICATION
AND LEARNING

Wisdom allows us to see the truth and to make good choices. With wisdom we gain insights into how life works, what life means and how we should conduct ourselves while we live. Wisdom helps us achieve, grow and develop both personally and collectively as families, communities, organisations and societies. Communication is key for successful relationships and collaboration. We cannot relate, nor fulfil many of our social and psychological needs without it. Information and learning are the life-blood of change. We must be able to learn and to adapt in order to survive and to flourish. Communication is necessary to help us resolve conflict, to solve problems, to achieve goals and to implement strategy. All of these are necessary components of a happy, full and productive life. The quotes and reflections in this section are focused on topics such as listening, silence, sharing, learning, knowledge and wisdom, flexibility, patience, mistakes, diversity and change.

> In order to improve the mind,
> we ought less to learn, than
> to contemplate.

Rene Descartes, French mathematician and philosopher
(1596 – 1650)

We already know a great deal of what we need to know. As we develop, we actually un-wrap our Self. We un-fold and uncover the knowledge, wisdom, beauty and wonder that is already there. We are frequently constrained by our expectations, and by our self-doubts and fears. As we develop, we unwrap the magnificent being inside us waiting to be set free. In order to improve our minds, we do not necessarily need to learn more facts and figures. We often simply need to access what we already know, think and feel.

I develop, unwrap and uncover the knowledge,
wisdom, beauty and wonder in me.

> The reason we have two ears and only one mouth, is that we may hear more and speak less.

Zeno, Greek philosopher (335 BC – 264 BC)

Most people assume that communication is easy, natural and almost effortless. That is why it frequently does not work. True communication is more than the transmission of information. It is a communion with another. Communication, therefore, implies relationship. As with successful relationships, successful communication requires listening, attention, effort and discipline. Listening is a gift we give to ourselves and to another.

I can listen. I can intimately communicate and share with another, if and when I so choose.

> ## The mind is slow to unlearn what it learnt early.

Seneca, Roman playwright, philosopher and statesman
(3 BC – 65 AD)

Habits, and mind-sets are difficult to change. They are even more difficult to change if they were learned early in life during certain critical periods of development. Consider our vocal accents for example. The accent we spoke with when we were somewhere around ten or twelve years old will very likely stay our predominant vocal accent for life. We can soften an accent or learn to take on new accents, but this is a difficult and slow process. In the same way, what our parents, siblings, extended family, teachers and friends taught us when we were young, has become embedded in our minds and is difficult to change. If you are trying to unlearn a long-held, deeply imprinted pattern, be patient, it will be a slow process.

I am flexible. I can learn, unlearn and change.
I am also patient and I give my Self the time it
needs to adjust.

> **Be not ashamed of mistakes and thus make them crimes.**

Confucius, Chinese philosopher and reformer
(551 BC – 479 BC)

In order to learn, to innovate and to grow, we must make mistakes. In our work lives, we know that not all innovation succeeds. Venture capitalists expect only one in ten new ventures to succeed. In order to learn what will and will not work we pilot-test new processes and we prototype new products. In our personal lives we must do the same. We must try different foods, different places, different experiences; we must try different responses, thoughts, actions and ways of being so we can learn what works and does not work. Along the way, we will make mistakes. These mistakes are not bad. They are not punishable failures and crimes. Our mistakes are the evidence of our willingness to be flexible, to learn, to grow and to change.

I am not ashamed of my mistakes as they are evidence of my courage and my willingness to try new things. I am flexible. I am able to learn, to grow and to change.

Persuasion is often more effectual than force.

Aesop, Greek slave and author (620 BC – 560 BC)

It is difficult to make someone do something they really do not want to do. While we can try and force someone to do something by making the alternatives unattractive or by exercising our power and authority, there are significant costs to doing so. When we use force, while we may get compliance with our wishes in the short-term, we are also likely to build resentment and to watch the initial compliance drop off in the longer-term. It is often more effective to use persuasion. Logical persuasion sometimes works, but often does not. Emotional persuasion often works better, but it must be genuine, truthful and sincerely done. The best way to bring about change in others is to change ourselves and thus to persuade by example.

I cannot force others to change. I can change my thinking, my attitudes and my behaviour and this is often most persuasive.

> **It is the mark of an educated mind to be able to entertain a thought without accepting it.**

Aristotle, Greek critic, philosopher, physicist and zoologist
(384 BC – 322 BC)

Many of us are aware of the importance and power of listening. Few of us are aware of the power of true consideration. When we seriously reflect on a perspective, and consider a position or a thought, especially one with which we initially disagree, we can often learn a great deal. We can gain great insight and empathy with another by doing this. While we do not have to accept or agree with this other perspective, position or thought, serious deliberation of it often leads us to greater understanding, acceptance and peace of mind.

I can contemplate a different perspective, position or thought, learn from it and gain a deeper understanding of others. I am at peace with difference.

> I approach these questions
> unwillingly, as they are sore subjects,
> but no cure can be effected without
> touching upon and handling them.

Titus, Roman author and historian (59 BC – 17 AD)

There are some problems that seem so big, and some injuries that seem so deep, that they cannot be thought about let alone discussed. We must remember, however, that if you cannot discuss it, you cannot fix it. There is no way to solve a problem or heal a pain unless the undiscussible, the unmentionable, is brought out from its dark hiding place into the healing light of day.

I have the courage to face what I need to face in order to heal.

Wisdom is supreme.

King Solomon, Hebrew monarch (~1000 BC)

Even his griefs are a joy long after to one that remembers all that he wrought and endured.

Homer, Greek poet (800 BC – 700 BC), The Odyssey

The power of wisdom comes from balance and perspective. Wisdom comes from the feeling mind and the thinking heart. When the spirit, mind and body are connected the seeds of wisdom are sown.

I think with my heart. I feel with my mind.
I am wise.

Time as he grows old teaches all things.

Aeschylus, Greek tragic dramatist (525 BC – 456 BC)
Prometheus Bound

When we are young, we do not always have the experience or the perspective necessary to understand many things. We must remember to be patient. If we think about something long enough the answer will eventually become clear.

I keep the bigger picture and the long term in mind and with this perspective all things become clear.

Hold on to instruction, do not let it go; guard it well, for it is your life.

King Solomon, Hebrew monarch (~1000 BC)

A mind without instruction can no more bear fruit than can a field, however fertile, without cultivation.

*Cicero, Roman author, orator and politician
(106 BC – 43 BC)*

Part of our 'instruction' is intellectual; it is our modern, school-based learning. What is also needed, and is often missing however, is our spiritual and physical 'instruction'. Too many hours in front of the television and too few hours spent connecting with family, friends, nature, and our hidden inner Selves, is often our modern lot. The life-long pursuit of personal growth and development is a worthy ambition. Learning is necessary for success.

I am able to learn in many ways.

> Put away perversity from your mouth;
> keep corrupt talk far from your lips.

King Solomon, Hebrew monarch (~1000 BC)

If you have nothing good to say, say nothing.
There is no value, and there is often great harm,
in complaining and being negative. 'Corrupt talk'
does not change anything about the object of
complaint and it is often harmful to the complainer as it keeps the complainer in a negative
state of mind.

I think and speak positive thoughts.

> He who knows does not speak. He who speaks does not know.

Lao-Tzu, Chinese philosopher (604 BC – 531 BC), The Way of Lao-Tzu

> Man's chiefest treasure is a sparing tongue.

Hesiod, Greek didactic poet (~800 BC)

In our modern world we are continually bombarded by noise and by inane chatter. Many people just talk to fill in the silence or to cover over their insecurity. Often it is better to listen more and to think more, and to speak less. As we grow more confident and aware of our Selves, we can become more comfortable with silence. The more comfortable we become with silence, the more opportunities we have to grow our confidence and our awareness.

I am comfortable with silence. I am comfortable with my Self.

> To know that you do not know it is the best. To pretend to know when you do not know is a disease.

Lao-Tzu, Chinese philosopher (604 BC – 531 BC), The Way of Lao-Tzu

The world of knowledge can be divided into three parts: (1) what we know, (2) what we do not know, and (3) what we do not know that we do not know. It is this third part, of which we are usually unaware, that often causes us problems. If we know that we do not know something, we are aware of the need to find the knowledge and skills from those who have them. Unfortunately, if we do not know that we do not know something, this lack of awareness can cause us serious difficulties. For example, if we do not know that every time we get scared, we become angry or aggressive, this unconscious behaviour can cause great problems. This is why awareness is critical.

I am conscious and aware of all that I do and all that happens around me.

83

> I have hardly ever known a
> mathematician who was capable
> of reasoning.

Plato, Greek Philosopher (427 BC – 347 BC)

Reasoning – good judgement, sound sense, sanity
- requires a thinking heart and a feeling mind.
Some of us are so stuck in our logical, mech-
anistic, 'mathematical' minds, that we loose the
ability to truly reason and to be reasonable.

I am wise. I have and use good judgement. I have
a sound sense of what is good and right.

> Don't give your advice before you
> are called upon.

Erasmus, Dutch humanist and theologian (1466 – 1536)

Advice is unlikely to be listened to or followed unless it is asked for. When someone is sharing their thoughts and feelings with you about a situation or a problem, they usually just want to be listened to and heard. If we give advice and try to solve the problem for them, they likely will not be receptive to our suggestions. The only time to give advice is when you are specifically asked for it. This is the signal that the listener wants our advice and is receptive to it.

I listen well. I reflect back thoughts and feelings to the speaker helping them gain insight and make up their own minds.

I am the wisest man alive, for I know one
thing, and that is that I know nothing.

Socrates, Greek philosopher (469 BC – 399 BC)

While self-confidence has many benefits, thinking
that you have the one and only right answer or cor-
rect perspective is the height of arrogance. Thinking
that 'I am right and you are wrong' leads to arguments
in families and to wars on a global scale. Historically,
humans seem to find killing each other easier than
accepting that maybe there are others who know as
much as I know, are as good and as right as I am and
are loved by God as much as me. No one person or
Nation has all the right answers. To know that compared to all that there is to know in our universe, I do
not know anything, is a humbling thought. It ensures
that we question even our most cherished assumptions and beliefs. It breeds wisdom and tolerance.

*I am aware of my importance and my
insignificance in the universe. I am as important
and as insignificant as every other grain of dust
and bit of energy in the universe.*

It is by doubting that we come to investigate, and by investigating that we recognize the truth.

Peter Abelard, French philosopher (1079 – 1142)

Curiosity and a mild dose of scepticism are valuable traits. We should not believe everything we see, read or hear. Especially in our modern, information rich world, it is important to remember that it is rare that we read or hear unbiased information. Anyone can write anything they want to and put it on the Internet. All newspapers and television news programs have a personal and/or a political bias. All books, including this one, have a personal and/or a political bias. We must explore, investigate and consider what we read and hear and in so doing, we can find what is true for us.

I am curious. I am sceptical about everything until I have time to consider it for myself. I recognise my truth.

> The nature of God is a circle of
> which the center is everywhere and
> the circumference is nowhere.

Empedocles, Greek philosopher (490 BC – 430 BC)

Paradox and contradiction are difficult for many of us to deal with. We like our world to make sense, to be ordered, understandable and predictable. Whether we like it or not, our world is more often paradoxical and contradictory. Our notions of God, for example, are often simplistic. What if God was a woman? What if we each were God? What if God was not even a person? What if God was a spark or a divine energy within each of us? What if God was a single point that was everywhere? What if God was nowhere? What if God was a thought we use to make ourselves feel better?

*I am able to think. Anything I can conceive
of is possible.*

> He is a wise man who does not
> grieve for the things which he
> has not, but rejoices for those
> which he has.

Epictetus, Greek Philosopher (55 – 135)

Most of us have a great deal for which to be thankful. If you are reading this you very likely have a comfortable house to live in and a car to drive. You are not likely to starve to death this year. You have access to clean water and descent medical treatments and facilities. While you may not have the ultimate house or car, and you may not be able to afford to go out to dinner as often as you like, at one point in time, just owning a house or a car was a dream. You also have many non-material things for which to be thankful. Every in-breath and out-breath, every sunrise and sunset, every joy and sadness, every second of our life is a gift for which we should rejoice.

I am grateful for everything in my life.

> **Rewards and punishments are the lowest form of education.**

Zhuang Zi, Chinese philosopher (269 BC – 286 BC)

There is no reason to ever hit a child. When they are young, they are not able to understand why they should or should not do something or why they were hit, so hitting does no good and does great harm. It is a parent's job to control their temper so they do not have to stike out. When children are old enough to understand why they are being hit, they are old enough to understand why they should or should not do something and, therefore, should not need to be hit. It is a parent's job to explain the world to their children.

I can control my temper. I am patient.

ACHIEVEMENT, GOALS AND EFFORT

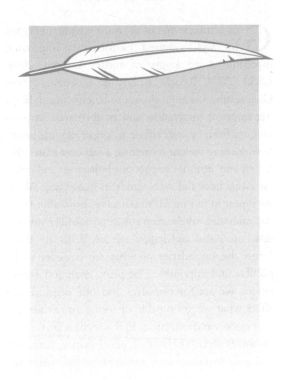

ACHIEVEMENT, GOALS
AND EFFORT

Goal-setting is one of the most widely supported and well-accepted performance-improving mechanisms we know of today (Latham, 2004; Locke, 2004; Roach, Troboy & Cochran, 2006). Goal-setting has been shown to be effective in helping improve motivation and performance in areas ranging from brainstorming to organisational profit, from loosing weight to getting a job or a mate. Our beliefs and attitudes impact our behaviour and influence our lives and our worlds in many ways. What we repeat in our minds to ourselves, hour after hour, day after day, week after week, profoundly impacts how successful and happy we are. What we think forms the boundaries of what we consider to be possible and impossible. The plans, goals and expectations we set for ourselves and our organisations affect what we are capable of seeing and achieving. The quotes and reflections in this section are focused on topics such as behaviour, performance, adventure and risk, commitment, accomplishment, planning, focus, patience, effort and persistence.

> Men acquire a particular quality by
> constantly acting a particular way...
> you become just by performing just
> actions, temperate by performing
> temperate actions, brave by
> performing brave actions.

Aristotle, Greek critic, philosopher, physicist and zoologist
(384 BC – 322 BC)

This reminds us that we bring into reality
through our actions; when we do something, it
becomes real. Therefore, we are limited only by
our beliefs about what is real and what we can
and cannot do. We all have an 'act'. We play many
roles. Our 'acts' define what is 'actual' or real in
our lives - how we are and who we are, and what
is possible or real for us.

I bring into my life all that I need through
my actions.

Great deeds are usually wrought at great risk.

Herodotus, Greek historian and traveller
(484 BC – 430 BC) The Histories of Herodotus

For many of us, we find that risk and danger are not at all exciting or fun. We, therefore, never seem to have any adventure in our lives. Adventure, however, is not necessarily always risky or dangerous. Adventure is action. When we make things happen in our lives, and become positive forces or causative agents, we are stepping outside of our every-day boundaries and risking ourselves, not necessarily by jumping off cliffs or out of airplanes, but by confronting and breaking through our self-imposed limitations. In this way, our lives truly become an adventure – a happening.

My life is an adventure … a happening.

> **The gods help them that help themselves.**

Aesop, Greek slave and author (620 BC – 560 BC)
Hercules and the Wagoner

> **Prayer indeed is good, but while calling on the gods a man should himself lend a hand.**

Hippocrates, Greek physician (460 BC – 377 BC)
Regimen

Meditation, contemplation and prayer are important in our lives. They are effective means of focusing our minds and of helping bringing forth changes in our lives. They are, however, passive means and must be supplemented by more active means. The yin and yang, male and female, inward and outward, and the passive and active are intimately connected. One is never as effective, or whole, without the other.

I pray and I do.

95

> If you aspire to the highest place, it is
> no disgrace to stop at the second or
> even the third place.

Cicero, Roman author, orator and politician
(106 BC – 43 BC)

In our modern-day, achieve-oriented society, it often seems that there is no place but first place. We seem to have forgotten that what is really important is learning, growing, developing and trying our hardest. One hundred percent commitment and one hundred percent effort are our goals. As long as we are stretching ourselves, whether we end up as first or last is of little consequence in the long run. It is the internal satisfaction gained from going beyond our limits that it is of long lasting value.

I live my life one hundred percent fully
and committed.

> Not snow, no, nor rain, nor heat, nor night keeps them from accomplishing their appointed courses with all speed.

Herodotus, Greek historian and traveller
(484 BC – 430 BC), The Histories of Herodotus

> It does not matter how slowly you go so long as you do not stop.

Confucius, Chinese philosopher and reformer
(551 BC – 479 BC)

When trying to achieve a goal, we often get frustrated or disheartened if we do not see quick progress and immediate results. We are often looking for the 'quick fix'. We want to lose weight in one week. We want to make $1 million overnight. It rarely happens that way. Studies and experience illustrate, however, that success is achieved and maintained by those who keep trying.

I am persistent. I will patiently achieve my goals.

> **It is easy to be brave from a safe distance.**

Aesop, Greek slave and author (620 BC – 560 BC)

> **Criticism comes easier than craftsmanship.**

Zeuxis, Greek painter (~400 BC) from Pliny the Elder, Natural History

Many people today would rather criticise than participate. From politics to sports to movies, we can solve all the problems of the world, moan about not scoring the winning goal and criticise a director or actor from our chair in front of the TV. It is much harder to do than it is to criticise. It is far easier to see how something does not work, than it is to go out and actually do it. Today, we need more doers and fewer back-seat drivers and critics. If you want to change the world, you have to do something about it.

I am a doer. I participate. I engage in life.

> **Give me where to stand and I will move the earth.**

Archimedes, Greek inventor, mathematician and physicist
(287 BC – 212 BC)

Nothing is impossible. Given an immovable place to stand, and a lever big and strong enough, we can lift any weight. A more modern version of Archimedes' quote is 'Whether you think you can, or think you can't, you are right.' It is hard to comprehend today that because most Europeans thought that the world was flat in the fourteenth century, it was then impossible to sail around the world - until someone did it. Until the 1960's, it was impossible to put a person on the moon. It was impossible to split the atom, to climb Mount Everest, to run a mile in under four minutes - until someone did it. It is now impossible to cure cancer, to travel faster than light, to feed everyone on the planet and to achieve peace on earth – until one of us does it!

I can do anything I choose to do.

99

> **A journey of a thousand miles begins with a single step.**

Lao-Tzu, Chinese philosopher (604 BC – 531 BC), The Way of Lao-Tzu

> **No great thing is created suddenly.**

Epictetus, Greek Philosopher (55 – 135)

Some goals or tasks seem overwhelming when thought about in total. They seem too big. They look to us like they will take an impossible amount of time. If we set smaller, more achievable sub-goals, or if many people are willing to do a little bit, we can often achieve amazing things.

I can achieve great things in small ways. I am willing to put in the time and effort necessary to achieve my goals.

> The softest things in the world overcome the hardest things in the world. Through this I know the advantage of taking no action.

Lao-Tzu, Chinese philosopher (604 BC – 531 BC),
The Way of Lao-Tzu

Giving in and letting go is sometimes better than forceful resistance. We all know that the mighty but rigid oak tree eventually breaks in the wind, while the soft and supple willow bends and survives. There is a time for strength, firmness and forceful resistance. There is also a time for submission and a time to give up the struggle and achieve by taking no action.

I am aware of when strength and firmness of purpose will help me achieve my goals. I am aware of when flexibility and stillness will help me achieve my goals. I am capable of either stance.

Haste in every business brings failures.

*Herodotus, Greek historian and traveller
(484 BC – 430 BC), The Histories of Herodotus*

**Celerity is never more admired than
by the negligent.**

Cleopatra, Egyptian Queen (69 BC – 30 BC)

In our fast-paced, immediate gratification world we must learn how to delay gratification. While it is difficult to balance near-term rewards with long-term goals, it is worth the effort. Studies consistently illustrate that people who can delay gratification (i.e., put off pleasure until their work is finished or wait for a reward), are more likely to be successful and more emotionally stable. They score higher on standardised examinations and have better overall grades. They are also more skilled at handling frustration and have more determination to overcome obstacles when pursuing a goal.

I can wait for what I want. I can work for what I want. I am determined and capable.

102

> **Force has no place where there is need of skill.**

Herodotus, Greek historian and traveller
(484 BC – 430 BC), The Histories of Herodotus

Frustration is difficult for many of us to deal with. When something is not working for us, we often have the tendency to push harder and to try and force it. It is often better to take a deep breath, to take a step back, to calm ourselves and then to apply skill and finesse rather than to try and force something out of frustration.

I am patient. I have the skills I need to make things happen in my life.

> Observe due measure, for right
> timing is in all things the most
> important factor.

Hesiod, Greek didactic poet (~800 BC), Works and Days

> It was built against the will of the
> immortal gods, and so it did not last
> for long.

Homer, Greek poet (800 BC – 700 BC), The Iliad

We must remember not to always force things. If we try something, and it does not seem to work, it is sometimes best not to force it. It maybe better to try it again later. The 'trick' is in knowing when you should or should not push through. If it is a self-imposed barrier, we must recognise it as such and apply all available force to break through. If it is a 'universe-imposed' barrier due to it not being 'right timing', then we need to recognise it as such and let it go for a while. Trust your Self – your thinking heart and your feeling mind – to know the difference.

I am sensitive to the will of the universe.

A nail is driven out by another nail.
Habit is overcome by habit.

Erasmus, Dutch humanist and theologian (1466 – 1536)

One of the reasons it is difficult for many people to break 'bad' habits, is because they try only to get rid of the 'bad' habit. It is difficult to put nothing in the place of something. It is more effective to replace a 'bad' habit with a 'good' habit. There are no prescriptions or easy answers here. You can replace smoking or over-eating with reading, walking, study, swimming, sewing, painting, singing or anything you can think of, but be sure to try and replace something that does not serve you with something that does.

I am able to change my behaviour.

Apply yourself both now and in the next life. Without effort, you cannot be prosperous. Though the land be good, you cannot have an abundant crop without cultivation.

Plato, Greek Philosopher (427 BC – 347 BC)

We must exert effort to achieve. For most of us, a life of silent, quiet contemplation is not possible or even attractive. But even an aesthetic or a monk's life requires great discipline and effort of will. In our modern world we reap what we sew, we attract what we focus on, we achieve what we work toward. We are the architects of our lives, laying every brick minute by minute, hour by hour, day by day, until we decide to move on to the next project.

I can focus. I can work toward my goals and achieve them.

> Concealed talent brings
> no reputation.

Erasmus, Dutch humanist and theologian (1466 – 1536)

While few people like a braggart, false modesty is equally dysfunctional. If you are accomplished and talented in certain areas, it is OK to be proud of the fact and to use that talent. Our world needs help right now. Do not be afraid to use all of the talent at your disposal to help make a positive difference.

I am aware of my strengths and my weaknesses. I am willing and able to use my talents.

If you wish to be a writer, write.

Epictetus, Greek Philosopher (55 – 135)

Practise what you wish to accomplish. If you want to be good at dancing, you must spend many hours a day dancing. If you want to be good at playing guitar, you must spend many hours a day playing guitar. If you want to write and to love, you must spend many hours a day writing and loving. If you want to make money and to have intimate relationships, you must spend many hours a day making money and intimately relating to others. There is no other way.

I practise what I want to accomplish.

> Nothing is more active than thought,
> for it travels over the universe, and
> nothing is stronger than necessity for
> all must submit to it.

Thales, Greek philosopher (624 BC – 546 BC)

Our thoughts create our realities and our futures. If we 'give-off' light and are positive in our thoughts and actions, we will attract bright, positive people, jobs, situations, and relationships to us. The law of attraction works. We create what is reality for us. Of course, no matter what we think, we are not going to be able to walk through a solid brick wall. In most aspects of our lives, however, we attract those things – people, money, employment – on which we focus. When we focus our awareness on some thing, even when we are not full aware of it, our thoughts and intentions have effects in the universe.

I give light. I receive light. I give love. I receive love. My thoughts and intentions reach all points in the universe.

> Hope is the only good that is
> common to all men; those who have
> nothing else possess hope still.

Thales, Greek philosopher (624 BC – 546 BC)

> Hope is a waking dream.

*Aristotle, Greek critic, philosopher, physicist and zoologist
(384 BC – 322 BC), from Diogenes Laertius, Lives of
Eminent Philosophers*

People need something for which to live. We
need goals, possibilities and things to look forward
to. Our dreams, hopes and aspirations create our
future. It is important for our mental health to
hope and dream.

*I am hopeful. I dream. I plan. I am optimistic. I
am full of hope.*

EPILOGUE

In unpredictable and highly contested environments, individual and organisational success requires the ability to handle stress and emotions, to adjust to change more quickly and effectively than your competitors, and to continually grow and develop your people and critical organisational resources and capabilities, while at the same time, running your short-term 'business as usual' (Turner & Crawford, 1998; Birkinshaw & Gibson, 2004). In order to do this, people need to be able to be in the present with clarity and power, they must envision and buy-into a potential future, and they must also deal with the past, emotions and the 'grieving' process some people must go through before they can let go and move on.

Change is an emotional process. People fear the unknown, being wrong, unaccepted, ridiculed, embarrassed and, therefore, frequently resist change out of fear. Many people have also become understandably cynical about change. We have seen management tools and techniques come and go by the dozen (e.g., TQM, BPR, down-sizing, out-sourcing, CRM) and have come to think, 'This too shall pass.'

I suggest that if we do not deal with this emotional legacy, we will continue to see slow or unsuccessful change. Not long ago, I conducted a 'quick-and-dirty' study of change practices. When I asked which one factor would help you most in your change efforts if you could do it faster, 15 of the 24 respondents (over 60%) answered overcoming resistance and building commitment. I also asked people to estimate the amount of time that was spent on dealing with the 'emotional side' of change (e.g., people's fears). On average, people reported spending about 13 days dealing with the 'emotional side' of change in successful projects, compared with 2.5 days in unsuccessful projects.

Fortunately, there is something simple that we can do to help foster a more functional emotional climate at work thus allowing people to deal with, and then let go of the past, while being able to focus on the present and work toward the future. The answer is to talk about feelings. We must allow emotions to exist at work. Emotions are normal and their expression is healthy. If you cannot talk about something, you cannot fix it. People need to have mechanisms for processing their emotions. This permission to discuss and process emotions is one of the greatest gifts that coaches and counsellors give.

Processing something is the exact opposite of suppressing it. Processing is the exertion of effort to facilitate the flow of energy. Processing means fanning the flames, fully experiencing an emotion or event, allowing the process of an experience full reign. In order to fully experience a problem we need to get it out into the light and into the open. We need to look the problem squarely in the face, confront it and each other's roles in it. Everyone needs to become aware that it is a problem and what its consequences are. People need to know what the alternative or desired state of affairs is, what the goals and vision of the future are, and how what is happening now and has happened in the past is counter to those goals and vision. Also, emotional support needs to be provided. Quite frequently, emotions are involved when a problem is suppressed. If emotions were not involved, the problem would very likely not have gone 'underground' and been suppressed in the first place. If people were able to fully discuss and confront the issues at the time, it would not have been swept under the carpet and continued to plague us.

In an organisational context, publicly acknowledging and fully experiencing a problem does not suppress the symptoms. In fact, it has the exact opposite effect. It certainly is not 'normal' or comfortable to do this at first. However, this allows the system, whether it be individual or organisational, to deal with the issues and provides the opportunity for cure. Of course, this works only with certain types of problems. Fully experiencing the fact that one of your machines has broken down, be it a computer or a lathe, will not help at all. However, this works quite well with non-technical problems (e.g., people problems and social-system problems).

The bottom-line, therefore, is that we need to encourage people to talk, and to talk about what is important, but not necessarily always comfortable. That means that we have to listen, not defend or justify – just 'shut-up' and really listen. This will allow people to process past experiences and emotions. It will allow people to 'get it off their chest'. This will allow them to begin to 'let go' of those feelings and the past – as all pain and hurt are in the past – and will allow them to begin to move forward. This may take a while and it will not necessarily be much fun at first. Once the air is cleared, however, you will see people more and more able to access emotion, express emotion, acknowledge emotion, release emotion, and move on (i.e., access, express, acknowledge, release, and move on). This will lead to quicker and more successful change, and to happier, more successful and less stressed lives. We fervently hope that this book will help in this process.

INDEX

action
    34,37,38,46,87,94,101
achieve; achievement
    v,10,31,58,70,92,96,97,
    99,100,101,106
adventure 92,94
advice vi,29,85
affluence 41
afraid (also see fear)
    62,107
aggressive 83
anger 36,42,48,60
aware; awareness – of self
    and others v,2,9–11,13,
    16,21,24–26,28,30,34,
    43,45,47,64,65,68,76,
    82,83,86,101,107,109,
    113

balance
    28,29,36,38,43,66,78,
    102
beauty 31,66,71
believe
    4,21,24,31,32,64,87
body 22,54–57,65,88

child; children
    13,51,58,90,
choice, choose
    2,4,7,21,24,26,29,30,
    37,47,60,64,72,99
comfort, comfortable
    8,82,89,113,114

communicate;
    communication
    v,15,59,70,72
conscious, consciousness
    2,5,9,11,14,17,21,24–
    26,28,30,34,47,49,53,
    65,83
create; creativity
    x,7,40,49,61,100,109,
    110
cure 65,77,99,114

death v,36,63,89
defend 114
difference, different
    14,18,19,47,74,76,104,
    107
discuss 51,59,77,112,113

education (also see learn)
    vi,76,90
effort
    v,7,12,72,92,96,100,10
    2,106,112,113
emotion; emotional
    x,2,33,38,48,65,68,75,
    102,111–114
envy 33
equal 67
exercise 22,38,56,57,61
excitement 45
expect; expectation(s)
    3,16,21,23,49,58,71,74,
    92

familiar 8
fear (also see afraid)
    11,19,63,111,112
feel; feelings
    ix,2,4,7,14,17,26,27,
    36–38,42,47,48,52,53,
    59,71,78,84,85,88,104,
    112,114
food 25,55,61,64,74
forgive; forgiveness
    36,38,40,48,68
friend(s), friendship 11–13,
    33,63,73,80
fun 58,94,114

give; giving
    2,3,5,20,26,29,43,72,
    73,85,99,101,109,
    112
goal(s)
    v,viii,23,43,44,48,70,
    92,96,97,100,101,102,
    106,110,113

happiness, happy (also see
    unhappy)
    2,6,21,34,36,38,39,63,
    64,70,92
habit(s) 30,73,105
heal; healing
    38,39,48,55,65,68,77
health(y)
    4,6,20,21,36,38,50,55,
    57,66,110,112

heart
ix,17,20,30,50,54,56,
58,64,78,84,104
hope 6,110
humor viii,59

impossible 44,92,99,100
influence 26,46,92
ill, illness 57
intimate 108

joke 59,60
joy 14,61,78,89
judgement 84

knowledge
44,45,70,71,83,114

learn; learning
v,x,2,10,11,13,19,23,33,
37,51,53,57,58,60,65,70,
71,73,74,76,80,96,102
lie; lies 36,54
listen; listening
57,70,72,76,82,85,114
logic 38,75,84
love 2,5-
7,12,13,15,18,31,32, 40,
46,57,61,64,86,108,109

material possessions;
materialistic 64,89
marriage 7,12
medicine 55,56
mind; mindfull
14,16,25,28,34,39,42,
54,56,57,59,61,62,65,
71,73,76,78-81,84,85,
92,93,95,104

music; musicians 61

neighbour 15,52

objective 24

pain 26,56,65,77,105,114
passion 33,36,45
perspective
14,24,59,76,78,79,86
persuade 75
poet; poets; poetry 45,61
possible; possibility
29,47,66,88,92,93,106
problem(s); problem
solving
21,26,28,59,65,68,70,
77,83,85,98,113,114
projection 53

reason 38,65,84,90
recreate, recreation
58,63,65
relationships
2,7,12,70,72,108,109
revenge 37,48
risk 92,94

secure 4,13
self; self acceptance,
awareness, choice,
expressions, love
v,ix,2,3,6,10,12,16,21,
22,24,25,28-30,32,37,
40,45,46,40,49,51,54,
64,67,68,71,73,82,86,
87,94,96,104,106
silence 64,70,82
songs 61

spirit; spiritual
2,8,10,17,22,38,45,54,
61,65,78,80
stability 8,51
success(full)
2,7,10,70,72,80,92,97,
102,111,112,114
submit

thankful 9,89
think; thinking
ix,2,4,6,9,11,17,24,27,
30,32,36-39,42,45,57,
71,75,78,79,81,82,84,
86,88,92,99,104,105,
109,111
thought; thoughts
ix,x,2,4,9,21,26,30,33,
38,47,55,57,74,76,77,
81,85,86,88,99,100,109
truth
24,31,42,54,59,67,70,
75,87

unconscious 30,49,53,83

wine 14
wisdom; wise
ix,14,30,53,57,78,84,
86,89
work
11,16,18,25,38,51,58,
63,72,74,102,103,104,
106,109,112,114
work-life balance
38,51,63
workplace v
words ix,x,14,21,31,39

Yin-yang 95

116

The Roots of Positive Psychology

For many decades, psychology has been dominated by a concern for the mentally ill. So-called 'abnormal psychology' and a focus on treating mental illness have been an appropriate priority. Recently, however, there has been increasing interest in applying what we have learned from the last 100-years of research and practice in psychology to the more positive side of our beings.

Two people have been extremely influential in this area: Martin Seligman and Mihaly Csikszentmihalyi. I recall reading Seligman's 1975 book on learned helplessness and depression (based on the work he and colleagues had been conducting since the 1960s on the relationships between emotions and learning) in graduate school. So when I heard about his book entitled *Learned Optimism* (originally published in 1992, now in its second edition 1998) I was pleasantly surprised. It was a revolutionary idea. For years I had been reading about and practising learned optimism and positive psychology and had not been aware of it. Csikszentmihalyi became well known as a result of his 1990 book on the experience of '*Flow*', the feeling we have when we are fulfilled and completely engaged in a task.

Seligman and Csikszentmihalyi seem to have legitimized the ideas of the personal growth and development movement, given them legitimacy and created an intellectual home. Arising from ancient shamanic practices, and reborn in the 1960s through drug-induced experiences, the quest for personal fulfilment and happiness now had a basis in scientific research and modern psychology.

James Carlopio, October 2006

Csikszentmihalyi, M. (1990) *Flow: The Psychology of Optimal Experience*, Harper & Row, New York NY.

Csikszentmihalyi, M. (1996) *Creativity: Flow and the Psychology of Discovery and Invention.* Harper Collins, New York NY.

Seligman, M. E.P. (1975) *Helplessness: On depression, development, and death*, W.H. Freeman, San Francisco CA.

Seligman, M.E.P. (1998) *Learned Optimism*. Second edition. Pocket Books (Simon and Schuster), New York NY.

Seligman, M.E.P. (2002) *Authentic Happiness: Using the New Positive Psychology to Realize Your Potential for Lasting Fulfillment*. Free Press (Simon and Schuster), New York NY.

James R. Carlopio, PhD

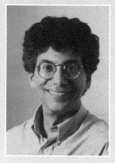 James Carlopio (BA, MA, PhD) has been a member of the Australian Graduate School of Management (AGSM) since 1990 where he has been a regular contributor to the executive education and MBA programs. James was the Director of the AGSM's Accelerated Development Program, a three-week residential executive development program for high-potential managers, from 1994 to 1997, and has been the Head of the Organisational Behaviour Group since 2005. His education has focused on psychology with a B.A. (Springfield, MA.), an M.A. (University of Manitoba, Canada) and a Ph. D. in Applied and Organisational Psychology (Old Dominion, Virginia).

James has worked on projects for numerous Australian and U.S. corporations, most recently in the areas of the implementation of innovation and new technology, organisational change, applying design principle and creativity to strategy design and development, personal change and influence, organisational and management development and strategy implementation and planning. He has worked with firms such as Rio Tinto, The ABC, Munich Reinsurance, ANZ Bank, Westpac, Vodafone, Telstra, Optus, SAP, AMP, NRMA, Commonwealth Bank, Deloitte Touche Tohmatsu, Applied Micro Systems/AAG Holdings/Volante, Australian Customs Service, Trowbridge Consulting, Australian Defence Industries, Mallesons Stephen Jaques, Honeywell Australia Limited, St. Vincent's Hospital Sydney, Austrade and The Pipeline Authority, in Australia, and with General Motors, Ford Motors and over 100 of their first and second tier suppliers in the U.S. During the past twenty years he has regularly conducted programs in organisational and personal change, strategy and technology implementation, creativity and strategy design, communication and interpersonal skills, and organisational behaviour.

James has published over two-dozen articles and three books on various socio-technical issues, and has written a regular section for the Australian Financial Review BOSS magazine. He has been a facilitator of short-term meetings and large-scale organisational change, and a speaker at numerous meetings on organisational strategy, cybernetics, human factors/ergonomics, human technology, and organisational behaviour.

From mid 2007 James will assume the position of Associate Dean (Executive Education), Director of the Centre for Executive Education, and Clinical Professor of Management, Bond University Faculty of Business, Technology and Sustainable Development, Gold Coast Queensland.

T - #0604 - 101024 - C0 - 150/104/7 - PB - 9780977574216 - Gloss Lamination